Breathe Brilliance

Unveiling the Marvels of the Respiratory Tract

By

Shirley L. Brooks

Table of content

Introduction

Take a full breath. Feel the surge of air as it fills your lungs, carrying life-supporting oxygen to each cell in your body. We frequently disregard a fundamental process that is as simple as breathing. However, have you at any point halted to ponder the complicated pathway that permits this trade of air to happen? Welcome to "Uncovering the Wonders of the Respiratory Plot," where we set out on an enrapturing venture through the sensational universe of our respiratory framework.

The respiratory lot, a mind-boggling organization of organs and tissues, fills in as our lifesaver, guaranteeing the conveyance of oxygen and the expulsion of waste gases. From the second air enters our nasal pit to its last trade in the little alveoli, the respiratory plot plays out an ensemble of capabilities that keep us alive and flourishing. In this investigation, we will uncover the mysteries of this surprising framework, diving into its life systems, mechanics, and the fundamental job it plays in our general well-being.

We will decipher the mysteries of each respiratory tract component during this journey. We will start with the nasal cavity and pharynx, grasping their crucial capabilities past simple air entry. We will then wander into the larynx and windpipe, finding the complex systems that safeguard our aviation routes and empower us to create sound. We will observe the remarkable process of air distribution and gas exchange within the delicate alveoli as we move through the bronchial tree.

However, our investigation does not end here. We will likewise dig into the mechanics of breathing, disentangling the planned endeavors of the stomach and intercostal muscles that permit us to breathe in and breathe out. We will come to an understanding of the regulatory systems that keep our breathing rhythm and depth constant and maintain a delicate balance between the supply of oxygen and the removal of carbon dioxide.

As we venture further, we will reveal insight into the different respiratory problems and infections that can disturb this agreeable ensemble. We'll talk about everything from asthma to COPD (chronic obstructive pulmonary disease) symptoms, causes, and the most recent advances in their treatment and prevention. We will stress the significance of proactive measures and early detection for maintaining respiratory health.

In our journey to keep up with solid lungs, we will uncover viable tips for respiratory well-being and support. We will investigate the job of activity, nourishment, and natural variables in saving the respectability of our respiratory framework. By understanding the effect of respiratory aggravations and contaminations, we can find proactive ways to defend our lungs and advance by and large prosperity.

At long last, we will look into the future, where rising advances and historic exploration hold the commitment to changing respiratory medical care. We will investigate the potential for imaginative medicines and avoidance systems that might change the existences of people impacted by respiratory circumstances.

"Disclosing the Wonders of the Respiratory Parcel" plans to motivate amazement and appreciation for the many-sided activities of our respiratory framework. By understanding its intricacy, we can engage ourselves to settle on informed decisions, focus on respiratory well-being, and esteem the breath of life that supports us. Thus, go along with us on this charming excursion as we leave for an investigation of the marvels that exist in our actual breath.

Importance of the Respiratory system

The respiratory framework is of foremost significance to our general well-being and prosperity. It fills in as the door for oxygen, the fundamental component expected for the endurance of every cell in our body, while additionally working with the evacuation of waste gases, like carbon dioxide. The importance of the respiratory system is highlighted by the following significant reasons:

1. Oxygenation of the Body: The essential capability of the respiratory framework is to supply oxygen to our body's cells. Oxygen is significant for cell breath, the interaction that produces energy for every physical process. Without a steady and sufficient inventory of oxygen, our organs and tissues would stop working appropriately, prompting extremely unexpected problems.

2. Expulsion of Carbon Dioxide: As our cells produce energy, they likewise create carbon dioxide as a side-effect. The respiratory framework proficiently takes out this waste gas, forestalling its aggregation in the body. Carbon dioxide, whenever permitted to develop, can prompt respiratory acidosis, a condition that upsets the body's pH balance and weakens ordinary cell capability.

3. Guideline of Corrosive Base Equilibrium: The respiratory framework assumes a crucial part in keeping up with the body's corrosive base equilibrium, otherwise called pH balance. By controlling the degrees of carbon dioxide in the blood, the respiratory framework directs the sharpness or alkalinity of our inner climate. This equilibrium is critical for the legitimate working of catalysts, chemicals, and other biochemical cycles.

4. Insusceptible Protection: The respiratory framework goes about as a protection system against unsafe microbes, contaminations, and allergens. The nasal hole and respiratory lot are fixed with particular cells and little hair-like designs called cilia, which help trap and eliminate unfamiliar particles, keeping them from entering further into the lungs. Moreover, the respiratory framework produces bodily fluid and antibodies that help kill and dispense with microbes, keeping our lungs and aviation routes solid.

5. Regulation of Temperature and Moisture: The respiratory framework controls internal heat levels and keeps up with ideal dampness levels in aviation routes. At the point when we breathe out, we discharge warm, clammy air, which forestalls over-the-top drying of the respiratory tissues. Because it helps protect the lungs' delicate tissues from damage, this function is especially important in cold and dry environments.

6. Discourse and Correspondence: The respiratory framework assumes a critical part in discourse creation. The larynx, ordinarily known as the voice box, houses the vocal lines that vibrate to create sound. By controlling the development of air through the vocal strings, the respiratory framework empowers us to make a large number of vocal sounds, working with correspondence and articulation.

Understanding the significance of the respiratory framework highlights the requirement for its legitimate consideration and upkeep. By embracing the solid way of life propensities, for example, abstaining from smoking, decreasing openness to contaminations, practicing consistently, and keeping up with great respiratory cleanliness, we can uphold the ideal working of this fundamental framework and advance our general well-being and prosperity.

Overview of the respiratory tract's components

The respiratory lot is a perplexing framework that includes a few interconnected parts that cooperate to work with the trading of gases between the body and the outside climate. Here is an outline of the principal parts of the respiratory parcel:

1. Nasal Cavity: The respiratory plot starts with the nasal hole, which is fixed with a clammy and slight layer of tissue called the respiratory epithelium. The nasal cavity fills in as the passage point for air, where it is separated,

warmed, and humidified before proceeding further into the respiratory framework.

2. Pharynx: Situated behind the nasal depression, the pharynx is a solid cylinder that fills in as a typical pathway for both air and food. It interfaces the nasal hole and the oral depression to the larynx and throat.

3. Larynx: Frequently alluded to as the voice box, the larynx is a design situated at the highest point of the windpipe. It houses the vocal ropes and is liable for voice creation. Furthermore, the larynx contains the epiglottis, a fold-like design that keeps food and fluid from entering the respiratory plot during gulping.

4. Trachea: The windpipe, usually known as the windpipe, is an inflexible cylinder made out of ligament rings. It reaches out from the larynx and branches into the left and right bronchi, which lead to the lungs. The windpipe gives a pathway for air to go through the lungs.

5. Bronchial Tree: The bronchial tree comprises an organization of fanning aviation routes inside the lungs. It begins with the main bronchi, which then branch into smaller bronchi or bronchioles, and ends in alveoli, which are tiny air sacs. The bronchial tree facilitates gas exchange in the alveoli and distributes air to various parts of the lungs.

6. Alveoli: The alveoli are little, grape-like designs situated toward the finish of the bronchial tree. They are the location of gas exchange, where carbon dioxide, a waste product, is exhaled and oxygen from inhaled air diffuses into the bloodstream.

These parts of the respiratory plot cooperate flawlessly to guarantee proficient gas trade and keep up with the body's oxygen supply. The respiratory system's overall health and functionality are influenced by the functions and adaptations of each structure. Understanding the life structures and elements of these parts is urgent for valuing the striking complexities of the respiratory plot.

Chapter 1: Nasal Cavity and Pharynx

The nasal pit and pharynx are two fundamental parts of the respiratory lot, situated toward the start of the pathway for breathing in air. Let's examine their physiology and anatomy:

1. Nasal Cavity:

Between the cranial and facial bones, behind the nose, is the nasal cavity, a hollow space. It is fixed with a specific respiratory epithelium, which is rich in veins and bodily fluid-creating cells. Key elements include:

- The Nasal Conchae: Three hard designs called nasal conchae or turbinates distend from the sidelong walls of the nasal pit. They increment the surface region and make choppiness in the breathed-in air, working with effective humidification, warming, and separating of the air.

- Olfactory Epithelium: The top of the nasal pit contains the olfactory epithelium, which houses the olfactory receptors answerable for our feeling of smell. At the point when airborne particles come into contact with the olfactory epithelium, they trigger the transmission of olfactory signs to the mind.

- Bodily fluid and Cilia: Cilia are hair-like structures made up of cells that produce mucus and line the respiratory epithelium in the nasal cavity. The cilia move in concert to move the mucus and trapped particles towards the pharynx, where they can be swallowed or expelled, while the mucus holds dust, allergens, and pathogens that are present in the air that is inhaled.

- The vessels: The nasal hole contains a broad organization of veins that help warm and humidify the breathed-in air. To ensure that the air reaching the lungs is at the ideal temperature for effective gas exchange, the air gains heat as it passes over the warm blood vessels.

2. Pharynx:

The pharynx is a strong cylinder situated behind the nasal pit and oral pit, reaching out to the larynx and throat. It fills in as a typical pathway for both air and food, and its fundamental capabilities include:

- Passage for Food and Air: The pharynx considers the section of air from the nasal pit or oral depression into the larynx, while likewise working with the development of gulped food and fluids into the throat, prompting the stomach-related framework.

- Tongue: The pharynx contains groups of lymphoid tissue called tonsils, which help safeguard against microorganisms that enter the body through the nose and mouth. The tonsils assume a part in resistant safeguard by delivering antibodies and invulnerable cells that assist with fending off contaminations.

- The esophagus: The pharynx houses the epiglottis, a fold-like construction situated at the foundation of the tongue. During gulping, the epiglottis deters entry to the larynx, keeping food and fluids from entering the respiratory parcel and guiding them toward the throat.

The nasal cavity and pharynx are pivotal parts of the respiratory plot, answerable for separating, warming, humidifying, and coordinating breathed-in air towards the lungs. Their multifaceted designs and works guarantee that the air we inhale is spotless, molded, and prepared for additional vehicles more profound into the respiratory framework.

Anatomy and structure

The respiratory plot is a progression of organs and tissues that cooperate to assist us with relaxing. It is broken up into two main sections: both the upper respiratory and lower respiratory systems.

The upper respiratory plot incorporates the nose, nasal pit, sinuses, and pharynx (or throat). The nose and nasal cavity channels, warm, and dampen the air we take in. The sinuses are empty spaces in the skull that assist in easing up the head and producing bodily fluid. The pharynx is a solid cylinder that interfaces the nasal cavity and the mouth with the larynx (or voice box).

The lower respiratory plot incorporates the larynx, windpipe, bronchi, and lungs. The larynx is otherwise called the voice box and contains the vocal strings that permit us to create sound. A tube of cartilage rings connects the trachea, or windpipe, to the bronchi. The bronchi are the fundamental branches that lead into every lung. Inside the lungs, the bronchi partition into more modest branches called bronchioles, which ultimately end in little air sacs called alveoli.

The alveoli are the practical units of the respiratory framework where gas trade happens. They are encircled by vessels, which permit oxygen from breathed in the air to enter the circulation system and carbon dioxide from the circulation system to be breathed out.

The whole respiratory lot is fixed with a layer of bodily fluid and cilia that assist in keeping it clean and safeguarding it from unfamiliar particles. The cilia are minuscule hair-like designs that move in facilitated waves to clear bodily fluid and catch particles out of the respiratory parcel.

In general, the life systems and construction of the respiratory parcel are intended to work with the trading of oxygen and carbon dioxide between the body and the outside climate.

Functions of the nasal cavity and pharynx

The nasal depression and pharynx assume significant parts of the respiratory framework.

The area behind the nose that filters, warms, and moistens the air we breathe is called the nasal cavity. It is fixed with particular cells called cilia, which trap and move particles like residue, dust, and microscopic organisms out of the respiratory parcel. The nasal hole likewise contains veins that assist in warming the air as it goes through, making it more agreeable to relax. Furthermore, the nasal pit produces bodily fluid, which assists with catching particles and soaking the air.

The pharynx, or throat, is a strong cylinder that interfaces the nasal cavity and the mouth with the larynx (or voice box) and throat (or food pipe). It fills in as a section for both air and food. At the point when we inhale, the air goes through the pharynx before entering the larynx and windpipe. The pharynx likewise assumes a part in our capacity to talk, as it contains the vocal strings in the larynx that vibrate to deliver sound.

As the air enters the respiratory system, the pharynx and nasal cavity collaborate to filter, warm, moisten, and direct it. They help to safeguard the lungs from destructive particles and guarantee that the air we inhale is of ideal quality.

Importance of proper breathing through the nose

There are several reasons why breathing through the nose is important:

1. Purifying and filtering the air: Mucus-producing cells and tiny hairs known as cilia line the nose, helping to remove pollen, bacteria, dust, and other harmful particles from the air we breathe. Breathing through the nose permits these designs to trap and eliminate these particles, keeping them from entering further into the respiratory framework.

2. Dampening and warming the air: The nasal depression has a rich blood supply and a huge surface region, which assists with warming and saturating the air as it goes

through. Breathing through the nose guarantees that the air entering the respiratory situation is at the right temperature and dampness level, which is significant for ideal lung capability and to forestall bothering.

3. Improving oxygen take-up: The nasal hole contains structures called turbinates, which help to build the surface region and dial back the wind stream, permitting an additional opportunity for the air to come into contact with the nasal covering. This considers better oxygen take-up into the circulation system.

4. Animating the development of nitric oxide: The nasal cavity produces nitric oxide, a gas that assists with unwinding and expanding veins, further developing the bloodstream, and upgrading oxygen conveyance to the tissues. Breathing through the nose takes into account the legitimate creation and usage of nitric oxide.

5. Proper development of the jaw and face: Breathing through the nose advances the right tongue and acts against the top of the mouth, which is significant for appropriate jaw and facial turn of events. It assists with forestalling issues like malocclusion and the improvement of a long, thin face.

In rundown, appropriate breathing through the nose is fundamental for sifting and refining the air we inhale, guaranteeing ideal temperature and dampness levels, upgrading oxygen take-up, advancing legitimate bloodstream, and supporting sound jaw and facial turn of events. It takes into consideration the proficient working of the respiratory framework and generally speaking prosperity.

Chapter 2: Larynx and Trachea

The larynx and windpipe are significant designs in the respiratory framework.

The larynx, otherwise called the voice box, is situated in the upper piece of the neck, between the foundation of the tongue and the windpipe. The vocal cords, which are responsible for producing sound when air passes over them, are housed within this cartilage-covered structure. The larynx additionally assists with safeguarding the lower respiratory lot by keeping food and fluid from entering the windpipe.

The windpipe, likewise called the windpipe, is a cylinder-like design that interfaces the larynx to the bronchi. It is comprised of rings of ligament, which offer help and keep the windpipe from imploding. The windpipe is fixed with ciliated cells that contain bodily fluid creating challis cells. Together, the cilia and bodily fluids assist in trapping and eliminating particles and microbes from the respiratory lot.

The larynx and windpipe cooperate to work with the section of air between the upper and lower respiratory parcels. Air travels into the larynx when we breathe in through the nose or mouth. From that point, it goes through the windpipe and into the bronchi, in the end arriving at the lungs.

The larynx likewise assumes a part in gulping. At the point when we swallow, a little cartilaginous construction called the epiglottis covers the kickoff of the larynx, keeping food and fluid from entering the aviation route.

Generally, the larynx and windpipe are vital parts of the respiratory framework that assist in guaranteeing an appropriate wind stream and safeguarding the lower respiratory plot.

Role of the larynx in voice production

The larynx assumes an urgent part in voice creation. It contains the vocal lines, which are slim, versatile folds of tissue situated in the upper piece of the larynx. The vocal cords vibrate when air passes over them, resulting in sound waves that can be modulated to produce various tones and pitches.

The course of voice creation starts when air from the lungs goes up the windpipe and into the larynx. The muscles in the larynx change the strain and position of the vocal ropes, permitting them to vibrate at various frequencies. The size and pressure of the vocal ropes decide the pitch of the voice.

The sound created in the larynx is then adjusted and formed by the designs over the larynx, like the mouth, tongue, and lips. These designs go about as resonators, intensifying and changing the sound waves to make discourse.

Other functions, such as swallowing and preventing food and liquid from entering the airway, are performed by the larynx. The epiglottis, a small cartilaginous flap in the larynx, helps to direct food and liquid into the esophagus during swallowing by covering the opening to the larynx.

In general, the larynx is important for speech and communication as well as for voice production.

Structure and function of the trachea

The windpipe, otherwise called the windpipe, is a cylinder-like design that interfaces the larynx to the bronchi in the lower respiratory parcel. It is made out of C-molded rings of ligament that offer help and keep the windpipe from falling.

The internal arrangement of the windpipe is made of ciliated cells and challis cells. On the surface of the ciliated cells are tiny structures resembling hairs called cilia, which move mucus and trapped particles up and out of the trachea in coordinated waves. The challis cells produce bodily fluid, which assists with dampening and safeguarding the aviation route.

In addition, the trachea is made up of smooth muscle fibers that let the diameter of the trachea change slightly to control airflow. The windpipe additionally has flexible connective tissue, which permits it to stretch and agree with changes in the wind stream during relaxation.

The fundamental capability of the windpipe is to give a section of air to go between the larynx and the bronchi. It assists with leading air from the upper respiratory plot to the lower respiratory lot. The windpipe likewise fills in as a defensive boundary, keeping unfamiliar particles and microbes from entering the lungs. The cilia and bodily fluids coating the windpipe help to trap and eliminate these particles.

Overall, the trachea is an essential part of the respiratory system that keeps the lower respiratory tract safe and ensures proper airflow.

Protection mechanisms against foreign particles

The respiratory lot has a few security components set up to prepare for unfamiliar particles and microbes.

1. Mucus and hair in the nose: The nasal cavity is fixed with small hairs called cilia, which trap huge particles like residue and dust. The nasal pit likewise delivers bodily fluid, which assists with catching more modest particles and microorganisms. The cilia move in composed waves to push the caught particles towards the throat where they can be gulped or removed through hacking or wheezing.

2. Sneezing and coughing: At the point when unfamiliar particles or aggravations enter the respiratory lot, the body's regular reaction is to hack or sniffle. These activities powerfully oust the particles from the respiratory lot, keeping them from arriving at the lungs.

3. Bodily fluid creation: All through the respiratory lot, bodily fluid is delivered to assist with catching particles and microbes. The bodily fluid contains antibodies and catalysts that can kill or annihilate these unfamiliar substances. The mucus and trapped particles are then expelled from the respiratory tract by the cilia.

4. Mucociliary lift: The cilia, hair-like structures of ciliated cells, line the respiratory tract. These cilia beat in facilitated waves and help to move bodily fluid and caught particles upwards towards the throat. The mucociliary escalator is a procedure that aids in the removal of foreign substances from the respiratory tract.

5. Alveolar macrophages: In the alveoli, the little air sacs in the lungs, there are specific cells called macrophages. Macrophages are essential for the resistant framework and are answerable for overwhelming and annihilating unfamiliar particles and microbes that arrive at the alveoli.

These assurance components cooperate to guarantee that unfamiliar particles and microorganisms are kept from entering the lungs, limiting the gamble of disease and harm to the respiratory framework.

Chapter 3: Bronchial Tree

The bronchial tree is a mind-boggling organization of aviation routes that convey air to and from the lungs. It is made out of the windpipe, bronchi, and bronchioles.

The windpipe, or windpipe, is a cylinder that interfaces the throat to the bronchi. It is fixed with ciliated cells and flagon cells that assist in trapping and eliminating residue and garbage from the air.

The windpipe partitions into two fundamental bronchi, the left and right bronchi, which enter the lungs. Every bronchus then, at that point, isolates further into more modest branches called bronchioles.

The bronchioles are little, thin cylinders that keep on spreading out into considerably more modest ways called terminal bronchioles. These terminal bronchioles at long last end in small air sacs called alveoli, where gas trade happens.

The bronchial tree is encircled by smooth muscles that assist in managing the width of the aviation routes. This considers the control of wind current during relaxing. The walls of the bronchial tree are additionally fixed with bodily fluid creating cells, which help to soak the air and trap any excess particles before they arrive at the lungs.

Generally, the bronchial tree assumes an essential part in the respiratory framework by moving air to and from the lungs and working with the trading of oxygen and carbon dioxide between the air and the circulation system.

Anatomy and divisions of the bronchial tree

The bronchial tree is a stretching arrangement of aviation routes that leads from the windpipe (windpipe) to the alveoli (small air sacs) in the lungs. It comprises a few divisions that dynamically get more modest in size.

The fundamental divisions of the bronchial tree include:

1. Trachea: This is an enormous cylinder situated in the neck and chest that interfaces the larynx (voice box) to the bronchi. It is comprised of rings of ligament to keep it open and forestall breakdown.

2. Essential bronchi: The windpipe isolates into two essential bronchi, one for every lung. Every essential bronchus enters the lung and further partitions into auxiliary bronchi.

3. Optional bronchi: Every optional bronchus supplies one curve of the lung. The right lung has three curves, so it has three optional bronchi, though the left lung has two curves, so it has two auxiliary bronchi.

4. Tertiary bronchi: Every auxiliary bronchus further partitions into a few tertiary bronchi, otherwise called segmental bronchi. These stockpile the bronchopulmonary fragments of the lung.

5. Bronchioles: The smaller bronchioles that result from the tertiary bronchi's branching continue to divide and shrink. They have no ligament in their walls, and their walls contain smooth muscle.

6. Terminal bronchioles: The bronchioles in the end partition into terminal bronchioles, which are the littlest of the bronchiolar divisions. They lead to the respiratory bronchioles.

7. Respiratory bronchioles: The bronchial tree's smallest airways, are involved in gas exchange. They have flimsy walls and contain alveoli.

8. Alveolar conduits and alveoli: The respiratory bronchioles lead into alveolar pipes, which further separate into alveolar sacs. The alveoli are small air sacs where the trading of oxygen and carbon dioxide happens between the lungs and the circulatory system.

The bronchial tree's divisions and anatomy allow for the branching and distribution of air throughout the lungs, ensuring that the alveoli can exchange gas efficiently.

Function of bronchioles in air distribution

Bronchioles assume an urgent part in the dissemination of air inside the lungs. Their primary capability is to control the wind stream and direct it to various regions of the lungs.

The bronchioles are more modest parts of the bronchial tree that need ligament in their walls and on second thought contain smooth muscle. This smooth muscle permits them to choke or unwind, controlling the breadth of the aviation routes.

By contracting or widening, the bronchioles have some control over how much air enters various pieces of the lungs. This is significant for guiding wind streams to regions that need more oxygen or for diverting air away from regions that might be harmed or aggravated, for example, during asthma or other lung conditions.

Clara cells, which are specialized cells found in the bronchioles, also secrete a surfactant that keeps the airways' lining moist and prevents them from collapsing. They additionally produce bodily fluid to trap and eliminate unfamiliar particles or aggravations from the air.

Overall, the bronchioles are essential for controlling airflow and ensuring that oxygen reaches the alveoli quickly enough to exchange gas in the lungs.

Role of alveoli in gas exchange

The tiny air sacs in the lungs called alveoli are where gas is exchanged between the lungs and the bloodstream. They are in charge of the exchange of carbon dioxide and oxygen.

The walls of the alveoli are exceptionally dainty, comprising a solitary layer of cells called the alveolar epithelium. This slimness takes into account the proficient dispersion of gases through the walls.

Oxygen enters the alveoli from the air when we breathe in and diffuses through their thin walls into the bloodstream. Simultaneously, carbon dioxide, which is a side-effect of cell breath, diffuses out of the circulation system into the alveoli.

The trading of gases in the alveoli is driven by contrasts in fractional strain between the air in the alveoli and the blood in the encompassing vessels. Oxygen moves from an area of higher fractional strain (in the alveoli) to an area of lower halfway tension (in the blood), while carbon dioxide moves from an area of higher fractional strain (in the blood) to an area of lower incomplete strain (in the alveoli).

There are approximately 300 million alveoli in the lungs, each of which provides a substantial surface area for gas exchange. This huge surface region, alongside the slender walls of the alveoli, takes into consideration the effective trade of oxygen and carbon dioxide, guaranteeing that oxygen can be conveyed to the body's tissues and carbon dioxide can be eliminated.

Chapter 4: Mechanics of Breathing

Mechanics of breathing alludes to the interaction by which air is coaxed into and ousted out of the lungs. It includes the planned development of different muscles and changes in strain inside the thoracic cavity.

The diaphragm and external intercostal muscles contract while inhaling, or inspiration. The stomach, a vault-molded muscle at the foundation of the lungs, straightens and moves to descend, while the outer intercostal muscles between the ribs agree and lift the rib confine. The thoracic cavity gets bigger as a result of these movements, which lowers the pressure in the lungs. Consequently, following the pressure gradient, air is drawn into the lungs from the atmosphere.

During exhalation or termination, the stomach and outside intercostal muscles unwind. The stomach gets back to its arch shape and moves up, while the outer intercostal muscles unwind, permitting the rib enclosure to lower. This diminishes the volume of the thoracic cavity, causing an expansion in strain inside the lungs. Subsequently, air is removed from the lungs and out into the environment.

The mechanics of breathing additionally include the extra muscles of breath, which can be enlisted during respiratory trouble or expanded respiratory interest. The scalene muscles in the upper chest, the sternocleidomastoid muscles in the neck, and the abdominal muscles are examples of these.

In general, the mechanics of breathing depend on the organized constriction and unwinding of different muscles to make changes in tension inside the thoracic hole, considering the development of air all through the lungs.

Inspiration and expiration processes

When air is drawn into and expelled from the lungs, inspiration and expiration are the two processes involved in breathing.

Motivation, or inward breath, is the most common way of carrying air into the lungs. It includes the withdrawal of the stomach and the outer intercostal muscles.

The external intercostal muscles contract, lifting the rib cage up and out, while the diaphragm contracts and moves downward during inspiration. These developments increment the volume of the thoracic pit, which prompts a lessening in tension inside the lungs. Subsequently, air from the climate is brought into the lungs, following the tension slope.

Termination, or exhalation, is the most common way of removing air from the lungs. It includes the unwinding of the stomach and the outer intercostal muscles.

The diaphragm relaxes and moves upward during exhalation, and the external intercostal muscles relax, allowing the rib cage to move inward and lower. These developments decline the volume of the thoracic pit, which prompts an expansion in tension inside the lungs. Subsequently, air is removed from the lungs and delivered into the climate.

Typically, during normal breathing, exhalation is a passive process that relies on the lungs and chest wall's elastic recoil. Notwithstanding, during expanded respiratory interest or respiratory trouble, the adornment muscles of breath, for example, the sternocleidomastoid muscles and the abs, can be enrolled to help with the course of lapse.

By and large, the cycles of motivation and lapse cooperate to guarantee the trading of oxygen and carbon dioxide in the lungs and keep up with satisfactory ventilation.

Role of diaphragm and intercostal muscles

The stomach and intercostal muscles assume vital parts during the time spent breathing by assisting with making changes in strain inside the thoracic hole.

The stomach is a vault-formed muscle situated at the foundation of the lungs. During inward breath, it contracts and straightens, moving lower and developing the thoracic cavity. This constriction of the stomach expands the volume of the chest, which prompts a lessening in tension inside the lungs. This abatement in pressure permits air to stream into the lungs from the climate, following the tension angle. During exhalation, the stomach unwinds and moves up, decreasing the volume of the chest and causing an expansion in tension inside the lungs, prompting the removal of air.

The intercostal muscles are situated between the ribs and have two layers: the outside intercostal muscles and the inside intercostal muscles. During inward breath, the outside intercostal muscles contract, lifting the rib confine up and out, which further builds the volume of the thoracic hole. This development of the rib confine assists with growing the lungs and reducing the strain inside them. The external intercostal muscles relax during exhalation, allowing the rib cage to lower. This makes the thoracic cavity smaller and increases the pressure in the lungs.

The interior intercostal muscles are engaged with constrained exhalation and assume a part in diminishing the volume of the thoracic pit by pulling the ribs descending and internal.

In a nutshell, the diaphragm and intercostal muscles collaborate to alter the pressure in the thoracic cavity, allowing air to be breathed in and out.

Regulation of breathing rate and depth

The rate and profundity of breathing, otherwise called respiratory rate and flowing volume, are directed by a few elements to keep up with legitimate oxygen and carbon dioxide levels in the body. The essential control of breathing is directed by the respiratory focus in the mind, explicitly in the medulla oblongata and the pons.

The medulla oblongata contains the essential respiratory focus, which produces the fundamental musicality of relaxing. It conveys nerve messages to the stomach and intercostal muscles to start inward breath and exhalation. The medulla oblongata additionally contains chemosensitive regions that screen the degrees of carbon dioxide, oxygen, and hydrogen particles (pH) in the blood. At the point when the degrees of carbon dioxide or hydrogen particles increment or the oxygen levels decline, the chemoreceptors in the medulla oblongata convey messages to expand the respiratory rate and profundity to eliminate carbon dioxide and reestablish oxygen levels.

The pons likewise assume a part in controlling the rate and profundity of relaxing. It contains the pneumatic focus, which conveys inhibitory messages to the medulla oblongata to direct the respiratory mood and forestall unreasonable inward breath. The apneustic center, which sends stimulatory signals to the medulla oblongata to lengthen inhalation and increase tidal volume, is also found there.

Other factors, in addition to the brain's respiratory centers, can affect breathing rate and depth. These include:

- Control by choice: We can deliberately supersede the compulsory control of relaxing. For instance, we can pause our breathing or control the rate and profundity of our breathing during exercises like singing or talking.

- Input from receptors: Receptors in the lungs, muscles, and joints give criticism to the respiratory focuses in the cerebrum, changing the rate and profundity of breathing to address the body's issues. For instance, to meet the increased demand for oxygen during exercise, muscle receptors send signals that prompt the respiratory rate and depth to be increased.

- Profound and mental variables: Feelings, stress, tension, and other mental variables can likewise impact relaxing. For instance, dread or frenzy can prompt fast breathing (hyperventilation), while unwinding or reflection can prompt increasingly slow relaxing.

By and large, the guidelines for breathing rate and profundity include a complicated exchange between the respiratory focuses in the mind, criticism from receptors, and different physiological and mental variables. As a result, the body can adapt to a variety of conditions and demands while also maintaining the appropriate levels of oxygen and carbon dioxide.

Chapter 5: Respiratory Disorders and Diseases

The lungs and respiratory system can be affected by a variety of respiratory conditions and diseases. A few normal models include:

- Earache: an ongoing condition that causes irritation and limiting of aviation routes, prompting trouble breathing, wheezing, and hacking.

- Persistent obstructive pneumonic illness (COPD): a dynamic lung sickness that incorporates persistent bronchitis and emphysema. It is primarily caused by long-distance openness aggravations, such as tobacco smoke.

- Pneumonia: a disease that aggravates the air sacs in one or the two lungs, making them load up with liquid or discharge. It can be brought on by fungi, viruses, or bacteria.

- Tuberculosis (TB): an infectious disease that mostly affects the lungs and is brought on by bacteria. When an infected person coughs or sneezes, it is transmitted through droplets in the air.

- Cellular breakdown in the lungs: a kind of malignant growth that beginnings in the lungs and can spread to different pieces of the body. It is typically brought about by smoking; however, it can likewise be brought about by openness to specific synthetic substances or hereditary variables.

- Thrombosis of the lungs: a blood clot that has traveled from another part of the body to block one of the pulmonary arteries in the lungs.

- Rest apnea: a sleep disorder in which a person stops breathing repeatedly while they are sleeping, resulting in disturbed sleep and low oxygen levels.

- Cystic fibrosis: a hereditary issue that causes the development of thick, tacky bodily fluid, which can obstruct aviation routes and make it challenging to relax.

- Pneumonic fibrosis: a dynamic illness that causes scarring and solidifying of the lung tissue, prompting trouble breathing and diminished lung capability.

- Rhinitis caused by allergies: an unfavorably susceptible response to airborne allergens (like dust or residue bugs) that influence the nasal sections, causing wheezing, tingling, and clogging.

These are just a few of the many respiratory conditions and diseases that can affect lung health and function. Looking for legitimate clinical consideration and treatment for any respiratory side effects or concerns is significant.

Causes, symptoms, and treatments

Depending on the condition, respiratory disorders and diseases can have different causes, symptoms, and treatments. Some general examples are as follows:

- Asthma: Causes can incorporate hereditary qualities, sensitivities, and openness to specific triggers like residue, pets, or exercise. Wheezing, coughing, chest tightness, and shortness of breath are all possible signs. Treatment frequently incorporates a blend of staying away from triggers, utilizing inhalers to oversee side effects, and taking meds to control irritation.

- Constant obstructive aspiratory illness (COPD): The essential driver is smoking, even though openness to ecological poisons can likewise contribute. Hacking, wheezing, windedness, and chest tightness are possible side effects. Pulmonary rehabilitation, the use of inhalers or other medications to manage symptoms, and quitting smoking are all parts of the treatment.

- Pneumonia: Bacterial, viral, or contagious diseases are regularly the reason. Side effects frequently incorporate fever, hack, chest agony, and trouble relaxing. Treatment might incorporate anti-infection agents, antiviral meds, or antifungal drugs, contingent upon the reason for the disease.

- Tuberculosis (TB): This bacterial contamination is spread through airborne beads. Side effects might incorporate constant hacks, chest torment, weight reduction, and fever. Treatment comprises a mix of anti-toxins taken for quite a long time.

- Cellular breakdown in the lungs: Tobacco smoking is the main source, even though openness to specific synthetic substances or hereditary elements can likewise contribute. Side effects can differ however may incorporate tireless hacks, chest torment, weight reduction, and windedness. Therapy choices rely upon the phase of the malignant growth and may incorporate a medical procedure, radiation treatment, chemotherapy, or designated treatment.

- Rest apnea: The most widely recognized type, obstructive rest apnea, is brought about by the unwinding of the muscles in the throat during rest, prompting halfway or complete blockage of the aviation route. Loud snoring, excessive daytime sleepiness, and gasping for air during sleep are all possible signs. Treatment options include using a continuous positive airway pressure (CPAP) machine and making lifestyle changes like losing weight and sleeping on your side.
- Cystic fibrosis: This hereditary issue influences the creation of bodily fluid and prompts repetitive respiratory diseases and trouble relaxing. Treatment incorporates prescriptions to clean bodily fluid off of the lungs, anti-infection agents to treat diseases, and treatments to oversee side effects.

- Aspiratory fibrosis: The reason is in many cases obscure; however, it very well may be connected with specific immune system illnesses, openness to natural contaminations, or certain prescriptions. Side effects might incorporate windedness, dry hacks, and weakness. There are few treatment options, but pulmonary rehabilitation and certain medications may help manage symptoms.

- Rhinitis caused by allergies: This condition is an unfavorably susceptible response to airborne allergens. A runny nose, sneezing, itching, and nasal congestion are all common signs. Treatment frequently includes keeping away from triggers whenever the situation allows and utilizing prescriptions, for example, allergy medicines or nasal showers to oversee side effects.

It is essential to take note that these are general models, and every individual case might shift. Talking with a medical services professional is urgent for an exact determination and a suitable therapy plan.

Importance of early detection and prevention

Early location and avoidance of respiratory issues and sicknesses are critical because of multiple factors:

1. Treatment adequacy: Early location takes into consideration ideal mediation, which can further develop treatment adequacy and results. Early detection of respiratory conditions can help slow their progression and stop further damage to the lungs, which is often the case.

2. Personal satisfaction: Early location and treatment can assist in overseeing side effects and work on personal satisfaction for people with respiratory problems. By tending to the condition right off the bat, people can encounter better command over side effects and have a more significant level of work.

3. Forestalling intricacies: Numerous respiratory circumstances can prompt confusion whenever left untreated or undiscovered. For instance, untreated asthma can bring about successive intensifications and long-haul lung harm. Identifying and dealing with the condition early can assist with forestalling these entanglements and diminish the gamble of hospitalizations or trauma center visits.

4. Cost-effectiveness: Early recognition and avoidance can be practical over the long haul. By distinguishing and overseeing respiratory circumstances early, medical services expenses can be decreased, as people might require fewer broad therapies or hospitalizations.

5. General well-being influence: Additionally, early detection and prevention have a wider impact on public health. By recognizing respiratory circumstances early and carrying out preventive measures, for example, stopping smoking or diminishing openness to ecological

poisons, the general weight of respiratory sicknesses on the populace can be decreased.

Counteraction of respiratory issues includes way of life adjustments and staying away from openness to realized risk factors. For instance, stopping smoking, diminishing openness to handed-down cigarette smoke, and wearing individual defensive hardware (like covers) in dirtied or dusty conditions can assist with forestalling the turn of events or movement of respiratory circumstances.

Standard check-ups and screenings can likewise support early location. For instance, routine lung capability tests and imaging reviews can assist with distinguishing changes or anomalies in the lungs, even before side effects are available.

In outline, early location and counteraction assume an urgent part in overseeing respiratory issues and sicknesses. They work on individual results as well as broadly affect general well-being and medical services asset use.

Chapter 6: Respiratory Health and Maintenance

Respiratory wellbeing and support include doing whatever it takes to keep your lungs and respiratory framework looking great. Here are a few key practices:

1. Abstain from smoking and openness to handed-down cigarette smoke: The majority of respiratory diseases, such as COPD and lung cancer, are brought on by smoking. Assuming you smoke, stopping is the smartest course of action for your respiratory well-being. Furthermore, attempt to stay away from where others are smoking to decrease your openness to handed-down cigarette smoke.

2. Protect yourself from pollutants in the environment: Contamination, both indoors and outside, can adversely affect respiratory wellbeing. Do whatever it takes to decrease your openness to contaminations by keeping away from regions with weighty air contamination, involving air purifiers in your home, and guaranteeing great ventilation.

3. Remain genuinely dynamic: Normal activity can further develop lung capability and by and large respiratory

well-being. Participate in exercises that get your pulse up and build your breathing rate, like strolling, running, or cycling.

4. Practice great cleanliness: Clean up much of the time, particularly during cold and influenza seasons, to decrease the gamble of respiratory diseases. Keep away from close contact with people who are wiped out, and cover your mouth and nose while hacking or wheezing to forestall the spread of respiratory beads.

5. Receive an immunization shot: Respiratory infections and their complications can be prevented with vaccinations like the flu and pneumonia vaccines. Check with your medical services supplier to check whether you are state-of-the-art on suggested immunizations.

6. Keep a solid eating routine: A decent eating routine rich in natural products, vegetables, and entire grains can uphold respiratory well-being. Certain supplements, like nutrients C and E, have cell reinforcement properties that can safeguard the lungs from harm brought about by free revolutionaries.

7. Practice great indoor air quality: Keep your home very much ventilated and liberated from allergens, for example, residue and pet dander, which can set off respiratory side effects. Change air channels consistently and consider utilizing a humidifier if the air is excessively dry.

8. Make sure you practice proper breathing: Profound breathing activities and strategies, for example, pressed together lip breathing and diaphragmatic breathing, can assist with further developing lung limits and diminish windedness.

9. Oversee pressure: Stress and nervousness can add to respiratory side effects like windedness. Practice

pressure-the-board procedures, like profound breathing activities, reflection, or yoga, to help unwind and work on respiratory well-being.

10. Standard check-ups and screenings: Ordinary visits to your medical care supplier can assist with identifying any early indications of respiratory issues. At the point when suitable, your medical care supplier might suggest lung capability tests or imaging reviews to evaluate your respiratory well-being.

You can maintain good respiratory health and lower your risk of developing respiratory disorders or complications by following these practices. If you have any worries or side effects connected with your respiratory wellbeing, it is vital to talk with a medical care proficient for a precise conclusion and suitable therapy.

Tips for maintaining a healthy respiratory system

1. Try not to smoke or stop smoking: Smoking is the main source of respiratory illnesses like the cellular breakdown in the lungs, ongoing obstructive pneumonic sickness (COPD), and lung diseases. Stopping smoking is the most ideal course of action for your respiratory well-being.

2. Keep away from openness to poisons: Attempt to limit your openness to air contaminations like handed-down cigarette smoke, outside poisons, and hurtful synthetic compounds. Use air purifiers and keep up with great ventilation in your living and working spaces.

3. Work out consistently: Standard actual work further develops lung capability and reinforces the respiratory muscles. Participate in exercises like strolling, running, cycling, or swimming to keep your respiratory framework sound.

4. Keep a solid weight: Obesity can make breathing difficult and strain the respiratory system. Through regular exercise and a well-balanced diet, you can keep your weight in check.

5. Remain hydrated: Drinking sufficient water helps keep your respiratory framework damp and forestalls dryness. It likewise diminishes bodily fluid, making it more straightforward to clear from your aviation routes.

6. Practice great cleanliness: Clean up regularly, particularly during cold and influenza seasons, to decrease the gamble of respiratory diseases. Cover your mouth and nose while hacking or wheezing to forestall the spread of microbes.

7. Receive an immunization shot: Keep up with vaccinations, especially for respiratory illnesses like pneumonia and influenza. Respiratory infections can be prevented and their severity reduced with vaccinations.

8. Practice profound breathing activities: Profound breathing activities can assist with further developing lung limits and keeping up with respiratory well-being. Practice diaphragmatic breathing procedures routinely.

9. Keep away from openness to allergens: On the off chance that you have sensitivities, attempt to stay away from triggers like dust, dust bugs, pet dander, and shape. Use air purifiers and keep your living spaces clean to limit allergen openness.

10. Have customary check-ups: Visit your medical services supplier consistently for check-ups, particularly if you have a background marked by respiratory issues. Early identification and treatment of respiratory circumstances can forestall difficulties.

Benefits of regular exercise and proper nutrition

Normal activity and appropriate sustenance have various advantages for general well-being and prosperity.

1. Weight the executives: Regular exercise helps you lose weight and burn calories. Joined with a decent eating regimen, it can assist with forestalling corpulence and related medical problems like coronary illness, type 2 diabetes, and particular sorts of malignant growth.

2. Worked on cardiovascular well-being: By lowering the likelihood of heart disease, high cholesterol, and high blood pressure, exercise, and a healthy diet can improve heart health. It reinforces the heart muscle, further develops course, and brings down the gamble of blood clusters.

3. Expanded energy levels: The body gets the energy it needs to work at its best when it engages in regular physical activity and gets the nutrition it needs. Practice increments bloodstream and oxygen conveyance to the muscles, while a decent eating regimen gives fundamental supplements to energy creation.

4. Improved emotional wellness: Practice has been displayed to lessen the side effects of discouragement, uneasiness, and stress. It makes endorphins, which naturally improve mood, come out. Legitimate sustenance, including omega-3 unsaturated fats and B nutrients, additionally upholds mental prosperity.

5. More grounded muscles and bones: Working out, especially opposition preparing, helps construct and keep up with bulk. Additionally, it improves bone health, lowering the likelihood of fractures and osteoporosis. An eating regimen plentiful in calcium,

vitamin D, and protein upholds muscle and bone well-being.

6. Further developed rest quality: Sleep quality and duration can be improved with regular exercise and a healthy diet. Active work decreases nervousness and stress, advancing unwinding and better rest. Certain food sources, similar to incline proteins and complex carbs, can likewise help with rest guidelines.

7. Improved resistant capability: Practice and legitimate nourishment support a sound safe framework. Normal active work can expand the development of white platelets, which assist with warding off contaminations. Essential vitamins and minerals that help the immune system function are found in a well-balanced diet.

8. Diminished hazard of constant illnesses: Customary activity and a solid eating regimen can decrease the gamble of constant infections like corpulence, type 2 diabetes, certain malignant growths, and coronary illness. They assist with controlling glucose levels, further develop insulin awareness, and lower aggravation in the body.

9. Worked on mental capability: Practice and legitimate sustenance have been connected to working on mental capability and a diminished gamble of mental degradation. Actual work increases the bloodstream to the mind, advances the development of new synapses, and upgrades memory and fixation.

10. Extended lifespan: A blend of standard activity and a fair eating regimen can add to a more drawn-out and better life. It decreases the gamble of unexpected passing from constant illnesses and age-related decline.

In general, ordinary activity and legitimate sustenance are fundamental for keeping up with ideal well-being, forestalling illnesses, and working on by and large personal satisfaction.

Importance of avoiding respiratory irritants and pollutants

Staying away from respiratory aggravations and contaminations is vital for keeping a solid respiratory framework and forestalling respiratory illnesses. Here are a few motivations behind why staying away from these substances is significant:

1. Respiratory wellbeing: Openness to aggravations and contaminations can bother the respiratory framework, prompting side effects like hacking, wheezing, windedness, and respiratory diseases. Drawn-out openness can cause constant respiratory circumstances like asthma, ongoing bronchitis, and COPD.

2. Lung harm: Cigarette smoke and industrial chemicals, among other pollutants, can directly harm the lungs. This harm can prompt lung illnesses and weaken lung capability, making it harder to relax.

3. Sensitivity and asthma triggers: Allergies and asthma can be sparked by a variety of irritants and pollutants. In people with these conditions, they may aggravate symptoms and inflame the airways.

4. Risk of respiratory infections rising: Aggravations and contaminations debilitate the resistant framework and make the respiratory framework more vulnerable to diseases. Respiratory infections can also become more severe and last longer if they are exposed to pollutants.

5. Cancer danger: Certain respiratory aggravations and contaminations, for example, tobacco smoke and asbestos, are known cancer-causing agents and can build

the gamble of creating a cellular breakdown in the lungs and other respiratory tumors.

6. Long-haul well-being impacts: Drawn-out openness to aggravations and contaminations can have long-haul well-being impacts, even after the openness has halted. It can prompt super durable lung harm, decreased lung capability, and expanded endanger of respiratory circumstances sometime down the road.

7. Ecological effect: Not only is it important for one's health but also for the health of the environment to stay away from things that irritate the respiratory system and pollutants. Contaminations delivered up high can add to air contamination and environmental change, affecting the respiratory well-being of the whole populace.

It is essential to avoid smoking and second-hand smoke, use protective gear in work environments, maintain good indoor air quality, and be aware of potential pollutants in the environment to minimize exposure to respiratory irritants and pollutants.

Chapter 7: Future Perspectives and Advancements

With ongoing research and technological advancements, the future of respiratory health looks promising. Here are a few future viewpoints and headways to pay special attention to:

1. Accuracy medication: Personalized treatments for respiratory diseases are on the way thanks to advancements in genomics research. By understanding a person's hereditary cosmetics, specialists can foster designated treatments that are more powerful and make fewer side impacts.

2. Therapy with stem cells: Foundational microorganism research holds incredible potential for fixing harmed lung tissue and treating respiratory sicknesses. Specialists are investigating the utilization of foundational microorganisms to recover lung tissue and

further develop lung capability in conditions like COPD and pneumonic fibrosis.

3. Immunotherapies: Immunotherapies, like monoclonal antibodies, are being created to target explicit safe cells or particles engaged with respiratory sicknesses. These treatments can assist with tweaking the invulnerable reaction and decrease irritation, offering new treatment choices for conditions like asthma and immune system lung illnesses.

4. Telemedicine: Telemedicine has seen a significant rise in usage, particularly during the COVID-19 pandemic. Telemedicine permits patients to talk with medical services suppliers from a distance, disposing of the requirement for actual visits and decreasing openness to infectious respiratory contaminations.

5. Man-made reasoning (computer-based intelligence) and AI: Simulated intelligence and AI calculations can assist with examining a lot of information and recognizing examples and patterns in respiratory illnesses. This can help with early conclusion, treatment arranging, and foreseeing sickness results.

6. Wearable gadgets and sensors: The development of wearable devices and sensors has made it possible to monitor the health of the respiratory system constantly. These gadgets can follow lung capability, oxygen levels, and other physiological boundaries, giving important information to analysis and the executives of respiratory circumstances.

7. Novel medication conveyance frameworks: Progresses in drug conveyance frameworks are working on the viability and accommodation of respiratory meds. Inhalers with savvy sensors and nebulizers with designated drug conveyance components are being

created to streamline drug dispersion and patient adherence.

8. Control of air pollution: Endeavors to diminish air contamination and control natural factors that add to respiratory sicknesses are supposed to proceed. Stricter guidelines, cleaner energy sources, and public mindfulness crusades expect to further develop air quality and diminish openness to contaminations.

9. Patient training and self-administration: Patients can be empowered to take charge of their respiratory health by emphasizing patient education and self-management strategies. Self-management and early detection of respiratory symptoms can be helped by improved educational resources, mobile apps, and technologies for remote monitoring.

10. Cooperative examination and worldwide drives: Cooperation among specialists, medical care suppliers, and associations all over the planet is essential for progressing respiratory well-being. Worldwide drives like the Worldwide Drive for Asthma and the Worldwide Partnership against Constant Respiratory Sicknesses advance exploration, instruction, and strategy advancement to further develop respiratory well-being around the world.

Emerging technologies in respiratory healthcare

Arising advances in respiratory medical care are changing how respiratory circumstances are analyzed, observed, and treated. Here are a few instances of rising advancements in this field:

1. Telehealth and remote observing: Telehealth stages permit medical care suppliers to evaluate and screen patients with respiratory circumstances from a distance.

This innovation empowers patients to have virtual encounters with their PCPs, diminishing the requirement for in-person arrangements and further developing admittance to mind. Remote observing gadgets, like spirometers and oximeters, permit patients to follow their lung capability and oxygen levels at home and offer the information to their medical services suppliers.

2. Wearable gadgets: For health and wellness monitoring, wearable devices like smartwatches and fitness trackers are becoming increasingly popular. These gadgets can follow fundamental signs like pulse and rest designs, which can give experiences into respiratory well-being. A few wearable gadgets likewise offer highlights like directed breathing activities to assist with overseeing pressure and advance lung well-being.

3. Versatile spirometers: Conventional spirometry tests, which measure lung capability, are regularly used in a clinical setting. In any case, compact spirometers are presently accessible, permitting patients to perform lung capability tests at home. These gadgets are associated with cell phones or tablets and give moment results, which can be imparted to medical care suppliers for remote observation and the executives of respiratory circumstances.

4. Man-made brainpower (artificial intelligence): A lot of medical data is being analyzed using AI technologies to find patterns and trends in respiratory conditions. AI calculations can assist with foreseeing illness movement, streamline treatment designs, and further develop conclusion precision. Artificial intelligence can likewise be utilized to foster customized treatment calculations in light of a singular's extraordinary attributes and reaction to treatments.

5. Augmented reality (VR) treatment: VR innovation is being investigated as a restorative instrument for

overseeing respiratory circumstances. VR can be used to create immersive experiences that help patients relax and forget about their symptoms. It can also be used to guide patients through breathing exercises and physical activities in a virtual setting for pulmonary rehabilitation.

6. Printing in 3D: For respiratory conditions, customizable medical devices and implants are being made using 3D printing technology. This includes anatomical models for surgical planning and training, continuous positive airway pressure (CPAP) nasal masks, and customized airway stents.

7. Advanced mechanics helped a medical procedure: Mechanical frameworks are being utilized in a medical procedure for conditions like cellular breakdown in the lungs, considering exact and negligibly obtrusive systems. Improved visualization, increased surgical precision, and less patient trauma are some of the benefits of robotic-assisted surgery.

8. Astute inhalers: Brilliant inhaler gadgets are outfitted with sensors that track drug utilization and inward breath methods. These gadgets can give continuous criticism to patients, reminding them to take their medicine and guaranteeing appropriate methods. Information from savvy inhalers can likewise be imparted to medical services suppliers for observing adherence and therapy adequacy.

Arising advances in respiratory medical services can work on understanding results, upgrade remote checking abilities, and give customized care to people with respiratory circumstances. As these innovations keep on propelling, they can alter the administration and treatment of respiratory sicknesses.

Potential breakthroughs in treatment and prevention

There are a few possible leap forwards in treatment and counteraction in different fields of medical care. A few examples include:

1. Quality treatment: To treat or prevent disease, gene therapy involves inserting or modifying genes into a person's cells. It can give a designated and customized way to deal with therapy, especially for hereditary issues and particular sorts of diseases.

2. Immunotherapy: Immunotherapy is a sort of malignant growth therapy that supports the body's normal resistant reaction to battle disease cells. Late progressions in immunotherapy, like resistant designated spot inhibitors and Vehicle White blood cell treatment, have shown promising outcomes in treating different sorts of malignant growth, including already untreatable ones.

3. Accuracy medication: Accuracy medication plans to foster customized medicines in light of a singular's particular hereditary cosmetics, way of life, and climate. By taking into account these elements, medical services suppliers can give more customized and powerful therapy plans, eventually working on understanding results.

4. Computerized reasoning (man-made intelligence) in medical services: Man-made intelligence can change patient considerations and further develop treatment results. Overwhelmingly of information, simulated intelligence calculations can assist with distinguishing designs, foresee sickness movement, and propose ideal therapy plans. This can prompt prior determination, more exact treatment choice, and work on generally tolerant consideration.

5. Emerging disease vaccines: Fast turn of events and organization of immunizations are pivotal for

forestalling and controlling the spread of irresistible sicknesses. Effective vaccines against diseases like COVID-19 have been quickly developed thanks to advancements in vaccine technology like mRNA-based vaccines. Continuous examination means to additionally outfit these advances to answer future episodes rapidly.

6. Painless diagnostics: Progressions in analytic advancements are making it conceivable to analyze and screen illnesses without the requirement for obtrusive methods. For instance, painless imaging methods, like X-ray and PET outputs, give itemized data about organ capability and can help in early sickness location.

These potential leap forwards offer further developed treatment results, customized care, and better general counteraction methodologies in medical services. Proceeded with innovative work here are supposed to additional development medical services from now on.

Promising research areas for respiratory health improvement

Promising exploration regions for respiratory well-being improvement include:

1. Improvement of designated treatments: Asthma, chronic obstructive pulmonary disease (COPD), and cystic fibrosis are just a few of the respiratory conditions that are being studied by researchers for potential new medications and treatments. This includes developing medicines that improve lung function and address the diseases' underlying causes.

2. Undifferentiated cell and regenerative medication: Undeveloped cell treatment and regenerative medication

hold a guarantee for fixing harmed lung tissue and advancing lung recovery. Specialists are concentrating on the utilization of immature microorganisms to deal with conditions like lung fibrosis and emphysema, fully intent on further developing lung capability and long-haul results.

3. Respiratory diseases and precision medicine: The goal of precision medicine is to offer treatments that are tailored to each patient based on their unique genetic profile. In respiratory illnesses, recognizing explicit hereditary elements that add to sickness improvement and movement can prompt more designated and compelling treatments.

4. Respiratory infection anticipation and treatment: With the continuous danger of respiratory infections like flu and respiratory syncytial infection (RSV), there is a requirement for further developed counteraction and treatment choices. Scientists are chipping away at growing more powerful antibodies, antiviral treatments, and better procedures to control viral flare-ups.

5. Air contamination relief: Respiratory illnesses are significantly influenced by air pollution. Research endeavors are centered around creating methodologies to diminish openness to air contaminations, for example, carrying out stricter guidelines, further developing air quality checking frameworks, and elevating maintainable options in contrast to dirtying enterprises.

6. Computerized reasoning in respiratory well-being: Man-made intelligence innovation can work on respiratory well-being in different ways, including more precise conclusions and forecasts of illness movement, advancement of treatment plans, and better remote checking of patients with respiratory circumstances.

7. Ecological elements and respiratory wellbeing: To learn more about how the environment affects respiratory health, research is being done. This incorporates concentrating on the impacts of environmental change, outside air contamination, indoor air quality, and word-related openings on respiratory infections, fully intent on creating compelling preventive procedures.

By zeroing in on these exploration regions, researchers and medical care experts desire to progress respiratory well-being, further develop therapy choices, and lessen the weight of respiratory illnesses on people and networks.

Conclusion

All in all, the respiratory parcel is a staggering and imperative framework in our bodies that permits us to inhale and trade oxygen for carbon dioxide. It is a complicated organization of organs, tissues, and cells that cooperate consistently to guarantee our endurance. From the second we take our most memorable breath to each breath from there on, the respiratory plot assumes an urgent part in supporting our lives.

Valuing the miracles of the respiratory parcel includes perceiving the mind-boggling systems associated with the course of breath and the fantastic flexibility of our lungs. A framework has developed more than a great many years to proficiently move oxygen to our cells and remove carbon dioxide, empowering us to complete our day-to-day exercises.

Moreover, an enthusiasm for the respiratory lot reaches out to understanding the different illnesses and conditions that can influence it. From normal diseases like seasonal influenza and asthma to additional difficult circumstances like pneumonia and cellular breakdown in the lungs, the respiratory parcel is defenseless against a scope of dangers. By grasping the dangers, side effects, and treatment choices related to these circumstances, we can focus on respiratory well-being and do whatever it takes to forestall and oversee them.

Last but not least, recognizing the incredible advancements in medical research and technology that have improved our comprehension of and treatment of respiratory diseases is an essential part of understanding the wonders of the respiratory tract. Leap forwards in regions like quality treatment, immunotherapy, and regenerative medication offer expected further developed treatment results and better long haul the board of respiratory circumstances.

Lastly, taking the time to appreciate the wonders of the respiratory system enables us to better appreciate the gift of breath and the significance of respiratory health maintenance. It fills in as a suggestion to focus on taking care of oneself, look for clinical consideration when required, and support progressing research endeavors that mean additional development of respiratory well-being to help people and networks.

I'd like to remind readers to put their respiratory health first. Your respiratory framework assumes an imperative part in your general prosperity and personal satisfaction. The importance of respiratory health cannot be overstated for the following reasons:

1. A healthy lung function: You can ensure that your lungs are at their best by taking care of your respiratory system. This will permit you to inhale simpler, have

more energy, and participate in proactive tasks without encountering windedness.

2. Diseases of the respiratory tract: Numerous respiratory illnesses, like asthma, COPD, and cellular breakdown in the lungs, can be forestalled or better overseen through sound way of life decisions. By keeping a solid eating routine, practicing consistently, abstaining from smoking and openness to handed-down cigarette smoke, and limiting openness to air contaminations, you can decrease your gamble of creating respiratory sicknesses.

3. Further developed insusceptibility: Your immune system is also closely connected to your respiratory system. By focusing on respiratory well-being, you can reinforce your insusceptible framework and diminish your defenselessness to respiratory contaminations, like normal colds, influenza, and pneumonia.

4. Early location and treatment: Standard check-ups with your medical services supplier can assist with distinguishing any respiratory issues from the get-go, taking into consideration brief therapy and the executives. Respiratory diseases can be halted from progressing and treated more effectively when caught early.

5. Better personal satisfaction: Focusing on respiratory well-being can work on your general personal satisfaction. At the point when your lungs are solid and working ideally, you will have more energy, better perseverance, and work on mental prosperity. You'll have the option to appreciate proactive tasks, inhale more straightforward, and have a more noteworthy feeling of imperativeness.

Keep in mind, that your respiratory well-being is in your grasp. Find proactive ways to focus on your lungs, like practicing routinely, rehearsing great cleanliness, keeping a solid weight, and keeping away from openness to contaminations. Assuming you have any worries or respiratory side effects, make it a point to with your medical care supplier. Your respiratory well-being merits focusing on, as it is a significant part of your general prosperity.

Inspiring awe for the complexity and resilience of our respiratory system

Our respiratory framework is genuinely stunning in its intricacy and flexibility. How it easily does the course of breath, permitting us to inhale and live, is out and out astounding.

Consider it: Our respiratory system starts working every time we take a breath. From the air entering our noses to the trading of oxygen and carbon dioxide in our lungs, each step is coordinated with accuracy.

Our lungs, with their complicated organization of bronchial cylinders and air sacs, give an extensive surface region to gas trade. The cilia coating our aviation routes work energetically to clear away bodily fluid and unfamiliar particles, shielding our fragile lung tissue from hurt. What's more, when we breathe out, the stomach and intercostal muscles cooperate to remove carbon dioxide from our bodies.

However, it's not only the mechanics of our respiratory framework that rouse wonder. Its versatility is similarly amazing. Our lungs have a mind-blowing capacity to recuperate and recover. Our respiratory system puts forth its best effort to repair itself and restore normal function even when it is confronted with damage resulting from illness, injury, or exposure to harmful substances.

Consider the way that our respiratory framework experiences endless difficulties consistently - from air contamination to respiratory diseases - yet it keeps on carrying out its imperative roles. The air we inhale may contain microorganisms, allergens, and aggravations, yet our respiratory framework has inherent guards to avoid these dangers and keep us sound.

This flexibility is a demonstration of the many-sided plan and versatility of our respiratory framework. It helps us to remember the significance of supporting and focusing on our lungs, so they can keep on serving us well all through our lives.

In snapshots of wonder for our respiratory framework, we can foster a more profound appreciation for the supernatural occurrences that occur inside our bodies every day. We can be propelled to focus on respiratory well-being, doing whatever it takes to safeguard our lungs from damage and backing their ideal capability.

Allow us to wonder about the intricacy and flexibility of our respiratory framework, and allow it to be a suggestion to focus on it with appreciation and regard. All things considered, our breath is a gift, and our respiratory framework is the inconceivable instrument that permits us to live and encounter the marvels of the world.